Time Management

Time Management Techniques: Unlocking The
Secrets To Optimal Productivity And Success

(The Productivity Manual For Lazy People)

I0135878

Stanley Chamberland

TABLE OF CONTENT

Chapter 1: "Time Is Not The Primary Concern. It Is All There Is"

Ever felt as though there is not enough time in the day? Why do some individuals appear to accomplish more than others despite having the same 24 hours per day? The solution is efficient time management. What is time management then?

Time management is the process of organizing and planning how you will divide your time among various tasks, and if done correctly, you will find yourself working wiser, not harder, to accomplish more in less time, even when time is limited and demands are high. This appears dismissive and unworthy of learning at its most fundamental level, but what distinguishes successful people from unsuccessful ones is the ability to control their time – effective time management.

In addition, time management is the practice of organizing available time and regulating the amount of time spent on specific activities in order to work more efficiently. Some individuals find it easier than others to manage their time, but everyone can develop habits to improve their time management skills.

Time management is more about self-management than time management. We all have 24 hours per day, but it is entirely up to us how we spend them. In contrast to others, successful people are ten times more productive because they are aware of this and use the information with discretion.

However, by learning and implementing the self-organization and personal effectiveness strategies in this book, you will finally be able to overcome internal obstacles that are holding you back, and you will acquire the laser-sharp focus necessary to accomplish genuinely remarkable things. If you learn and implement the time management skills discussed in this book, you will be able to combine your own efforts with those of others and utilize your intellect to achieve a truly phenomenal return on your time.

Therefore, devote some time to this book and implement its advice. Learn how to effectively and creatively manage your time, and your small time investment will pay off in spades.

Defining and documenting your objective is the initial step in developing an effective action plan. According to a study from the Dominican University, those who write down their objectives are significantly more successful than those who do not. Not only will writing down your goals increase your likelihood of achieving them, but it will also force you to focus on the process rather than just the final result. This is especially helpful when trying to identify objectives that are vague, aspirational, unformed, or less significant. To create a plan, however, you must adhere to the SMART goals framework, which comprises the following elements: Specific, Measurable, Attainable, Relevant, and Time-bound (or punctual). By utilizing this framework, you will be able to eliminate uncertainty surrounding an objective and develop an action plan that outlines precisely what must be accomplished.

The truth is that large goals can be so overwhelming that people yield up before exerting their greatest effort. They may become stymied when it comes time to specify how they will achieve the intended objective because they are too focused on the objective itself. However, dividing a goal into specific milestones allows the goal-setter to concentrate less on the end result and more on each mini-goal as a crucial step toward achieving the overall objective. If you have a plan delineating what must occur, you are more likely to remain motivated and committed to the process.

Identify the necessary resources: An action plan that does not account for resources is merely a wish. Whether you are working on a solitary project or as part of a team, understanding the resources necessary to carry out your plan will enable you to make informed decisions regarding its execution. These resources may consist of individuals or knowledge, technology and software, cash, time, or space. These are also essential for a successful plan.

4. Evaluate and assign tasks judiciously: Planning is dynamic, and different approaches can assist in achieving various objectives. If you are beginning a new endeavor, you could begin by assessing your current position in relation to your desired destination. If you are attempting to solve a pre-existing issue, brainstorming may assist you in analyzing the circumstance and considering alternative solutions. Prioritizing each activity makes your action plan more practicable in any circumstance. If you are flying solitary, prioritization will be based solely on effort and impact. However, when working in a group, it is necessary to prioritize and assign tasks in order to evaluate progress and ensure accountability.

Continuous evaluation and assessment: Creating an action plan is necessary, but not sufficient. Therefore, agility is essential for long-term success. A successful plan is dynamic and will alter as your business and circumstances evolve. According to the World Economic Forum's Global Risks Report, technological and societal advancements are causing significant workplace changes. Even the ostensibly impregnable strategies will undoubtedly be affected by these modifications. Therefore, the best way to ensure that your plan is still effective is to evaluate it frequently. In addition to allowing you to measure your progress against each task or mini-goal, a continuous review also enables you to make the necessary adjustments to meet your evolving needs, those of your team, or those of your organization.

Planning enables you to distinguish between duties that must be completed immediately and those that can be completed later. To better plan things, you should construct a task plan in which you list tasks against the time allotted for each activity. Prioritize high-priority tasks first, followed by those that do not require immediate attention. Planning enables you to complete crucial and time-sensitive tasks well in advance of schedule. Plan your day, your week, and every aspect of your life. Those who follow a planned approach complete their task on time, as opposed to those who embrace whatever comes their way. Working for the sole purpose of working is futile. Planning gives a person a sense of direction at work and motivates him to complete duties on time. Detailed planning enhances your life holistically by outlining the steps you must take at work to achieve your goals and objectives within a specified time frame.

Chapter 2: Why Your Time Is Valuable And Why You Should Not Waste It

Time is the seemingly irreversible succession of events that occur from the past, through the present, and into the future.

A person exists in this world within a time frame that can be expressed in the same manner, as evidenced by the fact that you were not the same person ten years ago in terms of your appearance, knowledge, or experiences. Everything around you alters as time passes.

Even though it surrounds us, time is one of the universe's most mysterious entities, and the majority of us take it for granted.

Why is it so crucial? What considerations should everyone bear in mind when contemplating time? Time is important due to the following factors:

Everything has a finite lifespan

Time influences every element in the universe. Everything, whether a tulip, a person, or a star, eventually ages and decays. Even if the rate of degeneration varies, all material objects eventually degrade and perish.

2. Time is the most valuable resource because it cannot be replaced.

How will you make use of the time allotted to you? Due to the fact that lost time cannot be recovered, the answer to this query is crucial. Money is often regarded as a person's most valuable asset, and while it is essential because it allows you to purchase the things you want and need, you can also get your money back. However, time is an immaterial resource, and once it's gone, it's gone forever.

3. No one knows their remaining time

No one knows how much time they have, which is yet another reason why it is so crucial. No one can predict the future, and death can occur at any age and for any reason. Upon becoming aware of this unpredictability, it is possible that your lifestyle will change drastically.

The present is the only time we truly possess.

Humans are aware of the past, present, and future as three distinct time periods. The only time we have to work is the present, but we can utilize the past to learn from it and the future to prepare for it. Improving present-moment awareness and living in the now has positive effects on both mental and physical health, according to research.

5. Happiness is determined by how we perceive time.

How someone perceives the past and the future has a significant impact on their happiness and sense of well-being. Many individuals are preoccupied with the past or the future. We would feel better and more at ease if we could let go of the past and things that cannot be changed, and instead anticipate the future with optimism rather than foreboding.

The caliber of its management has a significant impact on one's life.

As Shakespeare wrote in "Macbeth," "Let every man be master of his time."

Effective time management allows you to maximize every minute, which can be beneficial at home or at work. Time management, not talent, is frequently the determinant factor between success and failure.

7. A relationship's success or failure depends on the amount of time invested in it.

The community plays a crucial role in the health and contentment of an individual. Whether it's a friendship or a romantic relationship, connection maintenance requires effort, and time is a crucial factor.

Healthy relationships need time to develop. The primary difference between a profound and meaningful relationship and a superficial one is frequently the amount of time invested by each party.

The amount of time you devote affects your abilities.

Even though the exact amount is currently undetermined, it remains true that acquiring abilities takes time. In the past, it was commonly believed that 10,000 hours were required to perfect a skill. The exact amount of time required depends on the individual and how well they manage their time, but in general, it pays off to put in the effort and practice a skill.

Time can both teach and cure.

In the midst of a traumatic event, the adage "Time heals all wounds" may appear to be untrue, but individuals frequently discover that it ultimately proves to be accurate. Sometimes, time is the only way to gain a fresh, healthier perspective on a problem.

A person is afforded the opportunity to reflect on what has transpired and gain additional experiences during that time frame. While a person may not be able to return to their previous self, time has allowed them to develop.

Chapter 3: Methods To Stop Wasting Time And Actually Accomplish Stuff

It is simple to procrastinate and spend an excessive amount of time on social media when a boss is awaiting your work. Then, after another week has passed, you realize that you have accomplished very little. Aren't we all alike?

So many individuals have failed because they were indolent and did not act immediately. Indeed, if you examine successful people, you will notice that they all have the ability to get things done, spend their time judiciously, and avoid wasting time on unimportant tasks.

If there are any secrets to effective time management, optimizing your time would be at the top of the list. But how do you do it? How do you maintain concentration when you are distracted? How can you prevent bouncing from one task to the next and ending the day with nothing accomplished? And most significantly, how do you avoid falling prey to social media's allure? I will explain how to overcome procrastination and devote more of your valuable time to productive work and achieving success.

• Concentrate on a single task at a time!

This would be the only remark I would make if this list only contained one item! One of the primary reasons we don't accomplish as much in a day as we would like is that we switch between tasks without completing them. We like to cover it up by claiming we're multitasking and are therefore incredibly productive, but we're just fluttering!

And switching between tasks is one of the most efficient methods to waste time. Why? This is due to two factors.

The first is that it requires time to become comfortable with a new endeavor. Approximately the first five minutes are spent determining exactly what we're supposed to do and getting begun. We expend more time in the warm-up phase if we constantly switch tasks.

Suppose you labor on a single task until completion. Then, you may spend five minutes in the warm-up phase. If you move back and forth seven times before completing this task, you will have spent 35 minutes warming up and warming back up to it. It's simple, and I've already done it! Time has vanished into thin air. It will take you that long to complete everything on your to-do list for today.

More than two hours have been wasted. Consider what you could do with an additional two hours.

The second is that it is simple to become distracted by something that isn't on our to-do list and won't help us achieve our objectives when we flit. Concentrating on one task at a time prevents you from becoming engrossed in an endless cycle of distractions until you realize it's lunchtime.

• Only open a single browser at a time

The first will benefit from this recommendation. We have multiple tabs and documents open at all times, which is one of the reasons we are readily distracted. You are deep in your tasks when you realize that you have new emails or social media messages. Alternately, an open document may serve as a reminder of additional tasks associated with it. You will be significantly less distracted and much more likely to focus on the current task if you close all windows and documents other than those required to complete the current task.

• Stop monitoring social media and email immediately upon waking.

Isn't it a fairly typical manner to begin the day? Check your social media accounts before your email inbox, or vice versa. This is almost surely the worst thing you can do, for many different reasons!

In the first place, monitoring social media and email is a form of procrastination. I believe it's quite common to feel overwhelmed by all the tasks you must complete upon awakening. Checking social media and email in the morning feels like a pleasant and secure activity.

Using social media and email to avoid work is also extremely entertaining. When you check your email and use social media, distractions are abundant. It is simple to spend the entire day coping with problems that arise in the morning. This means you will be unable to complete the activities you had planned for that day.

There are three considerations when learning how to use social media and correspondence. One is that you may leave them open all day, allowing them to distract you from your task. Even if they dislike it, most people find that the first few hours of the day are their most productive and creative. You'll waste a lot of time if you use them to monitor social media. It is preferable to monitor social media as soon as you feel a little fatigued. Most of your mental capacity has already been utilized.

• Check social media and email no more than once or twice per day

This is a game-changing innovation! It initially seems a little strange. Isn't this a bit strange? Constant connectivity is the norm. Do you need to check your phone whenever it chimes, respond immediately to emails, and be a slave to notifications? But if you want to be more productive, you should never conduct yourself in this manner! On the other hand, it is a surefire means to become constantly distracted.

Then you will have control over your social media and communications, rather than being their slave. Set aside one or two times per day for email and social media. There are numerous tasks to complete before you can declare it complete. Close all open sites and notifications as soon as you're finished.

Then, proceed to the next item on your list.

This is notably true regarding email. If you check your email "every time an email arrives," you will conclude the day with a mess of opened/unopened/actioned/not-actioned emails. This is how the majority of people wind up with a frighteningly large inbox containing a thousand unread emails!

Giving your emails your undivided attention for a certain amount of time enables you to effectively manage email by deleting, filing, and responding to everything in your inbox simultaneously, and concluding the day with a clean inbox (and a lot of smug satisfaction!).

I will not lie: not receiving notifications and only "checking in" once or twice a day requires a great deal of self-control. The amount of time you could save, up to two hours per day, is still worthwhile. It takes much longer to deal with notifications individually than it does to deal with them in bulk, but the tension reduction is well worth it!

• Disable your phone's notifications

This allows you to focus on one task at a time and only monitor your alerts twice or three times per day. If your phone continues to "beep," you will presumably check in at some point. In this situation, you could power off your cell phone entirely (or even move it to another room)! This is not a smart idea if you have school-aged children or a dependent relative. I am aware that not everyone is comfortable with this. You desire the ability to assist in an emergency.

In this case, you may wish to disable all of your social media and email notifications, including the sound and the number that blinks on your home screen. This is typically accomplished through the preferences.

You will be able to leave the sound on for emergency calls while avoiding distractions from social media notifications! A slightly more extreme alternative is to disable sound when working from home and instruct anyone who may need to reach you in an emergency to use the landline!

Chapter 4: Procrastination

Depression is another condition that can contribute to procrastination. When a person is depressed, they may experience feelings of hopelessness, helplessness, and a lack of energy, which can make it difficult for them to begin (and finish) even the most basic duties.6 Self-doubt can be exacerbated by depression. When unsure of how to approach a project or unsure of your ability to complete it successfully, putting off a task may appear to be the simpler option.

Disorder of Obsessive-Compulsive Behavior (OCD): Individuals with OCD tend to engage in a pattern of behavior known as procrastination. One of the reasons for this is that obsessive-compulsive disorder is frequently associated with maladaptive perfectionism, which can lead to anxiety about making new mistakes, uncertainty as to whether or not a task is being performed correctly, and concern regarding the expectations of others.People with OCD frequently experience hesitancy, which causes them to delay making decisions for as long as feasible.

ADHD: A significant number of individuals with attention-deficit hyperactivity disorder (ADHD) struggle with procrastination.8 When external stimuli and internal thoughts are so distracting, it can be difficult to initiate a task, particularly if the task is difficult or uninteresting.

Different Forms of Procrastination

According to the findings of a number of specialists, procrastinators can be classified as either active or passive.

Passive procrastinators put off the task at hand because they struggle with making decisions and carrying them out.

Active procrastinators are those who intentionally delay completing a task because they believe that doing so will allow them to "feel challenged and inspired" while working under duress.

Others classify the various types of procrastinators based on the following behavioral manifestations of procrastination:

Perfectionists are individuals who avoid doing things out of fear that they will not be able to do them accurately.

Dreamer: A person who avoids responsibilities because they lack attention to the smallest of details.

Insists that no one has the right to dictate how they should spend their time.

The worrier is someone who delays completing tasks out of fear of change or forsaking the safety of "the familiar."

The person who causes crises is a procrastinator who enjoys working under duress.

The overachiever is a person who takes on too much and struggles to find the time to initiate and complete tasks.

STUDY BY LISTENING

Do not rush out and spend a fortune on the first collection of motivational materials you discover. There are a number of low-cost options for acquiring the materials you need to motivate you to be the best business owner you can be. Try your local library, visit the local Public Broadcasting Station, ask a friend in your network to share the cost and materials with you, visit a used bookstore, or search the Internet for previously owned products. There is a good chance that you will want to experiment with a variety of techniques and products, so it is essential to avoid making large investments right away. Take your time and investigate your options to ensure that you discover the most motivating material for your home business.

STAY POSITIVE

You must implement what you have learned to advance your home business. If you use the inspiration you receive to drive your business, you will rapidly start to see results.

Motivation can help you advance in both business and life. Consider what motivates you, and use what you learn from these techniques to refine your focus and reignite your passion for your business. Motivation can help you get started, but it is ultimately your responsibility to complete the task at hand.

Chapter 3 Reduce Your Clutter

We can only accomplish limited duties per day. We have unlimited options but limited resources. We must make important decisions in order to remove certain items. We acknowledge this when we feel incredibly occupied and superhuman. However, we cannot do everything. We must clean up the muddle.

Clutter is anything that prevents us from living the life we desire. It prevents us from accomplishing what is most essential. The frivolous items amuse us but do not advance our cause. They must be deleted as well.

The things that are most important to you will determine your decisions and how you spend the majority of your time. Why continue with a path if you are unsure of your destination? When developing a strategy, you must first determine your objectives and the guiding principles you will follow.

After defining your objective, you can begin to consider how you will achieve it. It is essential to establish your objectives. However, if you do not take the next step and formulate a strategy for achieving them, they will remain fantasies.

You must plan your journey to your destination. You must determine the most efficient means of achieving your goals. You must determine the necessary actions and resources. If we do not, we risk becoming enslaved by our environment and drifting through existence.

Knowing what to do is not sufficient. You must also have a firm understanding of what is not required. We have already determined that time is running out. We must determine how we will devote all of our time. In order to say "yes" to certain things, we will have to say "no" to others.

We will inevitably encounter circumstances that will cause us to abdicate our objectives. Sometimes, these impediments are caused by unhealthy behaviors. They are occasionally generated by those who wish for us to lose. They can also be triggered by less-than-ideal positive factors.

Regardless of the origin of the obstacles, we must pay close attention to each one and determine which activities must be eliminated!

Examine yourself to determine what makes you tick. What makes you come alive? What makes you feel alive and convinces you that you are not a checkbook-carrying automaton? What makes you feel emotional? What motivates you to prioritize the aforementioned things?

It could be listening to music, writing, singing, painting, dancing, sprinting, or lifting weights, among other activities.

3.1 The Focus Method
Time is something that can never be recovered. The Bible speaks of "redeeming the time" or "making the

best use of time." We have no idea how long we will remain on this planet. Therefore, we should capitalize on the opportunity. As we are continuously bombarded with interruptions, genuine needs, and distractions, we must commit to enhancing our organizational abilities.

We have lengthy to-do lists, far more than we can complete. However, it is far too easy to squander time. It is all too common to get caught up in the frenzy of activity, only to realize at the end of the day that our goals were not met. The desire to put off our most difficult but indispensable tasks is strong. In conclusion, it is a significant challenge to utilize our time judiciously on a daily basis, prioritize our tasks, and find a way to maintain a healthy balance between the numerous responsibilities, activities, and people we encounter each day.

The majority of books on time management aim to teach you how to organize your tasks and schedule so that you can accomplish everything on your to-do list. That strategy is impractical. You run the risk of burning out and exploding if you endeavor to do everything, which is counterproductive!

The first step is to acknowledge that you will not be able to complete everything. This implies that you will let go of a few items, decline a few requests, decline some projects, and reduce your to-do list. To complete the most essential duties, you will need to establish goals and devote the majority of your attention and effort to them.

Examine what you are currently focusing your energy on and what will be a waste of time as the first step in completing the appropriate tasks. This involves examining your overall life plan and being specific about your primary objectives and aims. As it will serve as the foundation for your daily, monthly, and annual goals and plans, you must initially devote a significant quantity of time and effort to this.

In general, you should establish your primary objectives for the year, also known as your areas of concentration. There will likely be a few categories for work and a few for personal life. You will be unable to keep up with too many attention areas if you select too many. As you organize your daily, monthly, and recurring tasks, it is advantageous to invest a great deal of your identity in certain areas of focus. This will help you align your daily activities with your ultimate professional and personal goals.

If you want to be a maestro of time management, you must identify what slows you down. Every day, we are inundated with interruptions, not to mention the wide array of time wasters and diversions that technology provides. How do you enjoy wasting time? Is Facebook at fault? Television? Or YouTube? Utilizing social networks throughout the day and night? What about computer games? Perhaps cooking programs? Keeping note of sporting events and their outcomes? Randomly exploring the web? Are you curious about celebrity news? The list could be endless.

Chapter 5: Skills In Emotional Management

What do emotional management techniques entail?

You can manage your emotional responses to events through the application of emotional management skills. They are a crucial aspect of emotional intelligence, which is the capacity to perceive and comprehend one's own and others' emotions. Although they may require some time and effort to acquire, emotional management skills can help you become a productive, professional, and supportive colleague.

Emotional control abilities are essential.

Initially, self-awareness

Self-awareness is a skill that enables you to anticipate how a situation or person may influence you by recognizing your emotional state. You can use it to monitor your emotional responses to situations and develop more effective responses. If you know that being prepared makes you feel more at ease and confident at work, you may make every effort to be as prepared as possible for the workweek. If you feel secure in your workplace, your stress levels may decrease and your ability to adapt to changes or difficulties may increase.

2. contemplation

By separating the emotion from the situation, reflection enables you to comprehend why you felt a certain way in response to a particular event or individual. Consider if you disagree with their decision or if you feel anxious about missing the debate, for example, if you disagreed with a colleague over a decision they made while you were out of the office. Understanding the source of your emotions may facilitate agreement with your colleague.

3. Recognition

Understanding how to embrace your feelings without valuing them may help you respond rationally to situations that are causing you to feel a certain way. By acknowledging your emotions, you can often recover from an emotional response more rapidly and concentrate on the next task. By relating your emotions to those of others, cultivating self-acceptance may also contribute to the development of empathy.

4. Viewpoint

By placing your emotions in context, acquiring perspective may assist you in gaining emotional control. For example, if you're anxious about delivering a speech in front of an audience, you can place this feeling in perspective by realizing that many successful professionals also feel this way. Perspective may remind you that emotions are a normal response to circumstances and that you can overcome them to fulfill your responsibilities.

5. Compassion

Empathy is the capacity to utilize one's own experiences to comprehend how others feel in a given situation. Employing empathy at work may aid in fostering positive relationships with colleagues and preventing conflicts. Empathy may enable you to recognize when a colleague requires assistance managing their burden and to empathize with them when they are frustrated by a difficulty or delay. If you have an understanding of their feelings, you can work with them to find a solution to the problem.

How to enhance your capacity to regulate your emotions

Discover methods for expressing your emotions.

You can better manage your emotions at work if you express yourself freely outside of work. You may discuss your emotions with friends or family members over the phone, which can help you obtain their opinions or a different perspective on your experiences. If you are creative, you could express your emotions through painting, drawing, or writing.

2. Recognize your comfort zones

Self-awareness entails recognizing positive emotions and the contributing factors. By identifying the aspects of your employment that make you feel good, you can develop a strong sense of success at work, which can make you more resilient in the face of challenges. Consider compiling an inventory of your favorite aspects of your work and displaying it in your cubicle or office.

3. Allow yourself space

When you find yourself in a situation that elicits strong emotions, it may be beneficial to temporarily withdraw. By physically removing yourself from a situation, you can regain your composure and improve your ability to reflect. You can go outside, but you can also acquire space by going to the break room or water cooler. If you operate remotely, you may peek outside through a neighboring window. After gaining perspective on your emotions, you can frequently return to the problem with a level head and generate a solution.

4. Investigate mindfulness.

Mindfulness is a meditation practice that concentrates on the current emotions and sensations you are experiencing. The purpose of mindfulness exercises is to help you concentrate on the present moment without fretting about the past or the future. Mindfulness can help you find calm and perspective regarding your emotions and daily activities. Start your meditation practice by focusing for a few minutes each morning on your respiration and the sensations in your desk chair or car.

Develop your respiration abilities.

A variety of breathing techniques may help you calm down and gain emotional control when you're in an emotionally charged situation. By focusing on your breath, you can minimize the impact of the emotion on your body and mind, allowing you to complete your task or find a solution. When performing a breathing exercise, inhale and exhale slowly and deeply. A common breathing exercise involves inhaling for four counts, retaining for two counts, and then exhaling for four counts.

Record your emotions in a journal.
Keeping a regular journal may assist you in gaining a deeper understanding of your emotional responses and in mastering their management. When writing in your diary, describe how you felt that day and what circumstances led to your numerous emotional responses. Re-reading your journal entries can assist you in recognizing your typical emotional states.

You will be able to anticipate how you will react in the future based on these stimuli.

Consult literature and podcasts about emotional regulation.

Numerous books and podcasts offer techniques for enhancing emotional control, with a focus on mental health or productivity. In addition, they may provide you with information on the brain chemistry associated with emotional responses as well as other details that may assist you in understanding your emotions. These materials are frequently located in the self-help section of bookstores and online podcast providers.

Consider speaking with a specialist.

By learning effective emotional management techniques from a professional therapist, you can boost your productivity and create a healthy work environment. They could lead individual therapy sessions or facilitate support groups for a range of conditions. In a safe environment, seeing a therapist may allow you to convey your emotions openly, discover the causes of your emotional responses, and develop coping mechanisms.

Chapter 6: Utilize Time To Achieve Life Satisfaction And Happiness

When you are in a state of experiencing and thinking abundance, you will begin to observe positive outcomes. Why? Because the universe is now rewarding you with what appears to be additional leisure. But when you take measures to better manage your time, these healthy methods will help you generate ideas that will work to your advantage. Therefore, you'll be able to attend to every aspect of your life with the confidence and assurance you need, knowing that the amount of effort you've invested in your career is sufficient. This will allow you to focus on other aspects of your existence.

When you are able to nurture other aspects of your life, you will experience personal development. Never will wealth equal completeness. Wealth only affects one aspect of your existence. There will always be this unexplainable vacuum within you, even if it affords you the opportunity to acquire a vast quantity of possessions. You are aware that it cannot be adequately fed with money alone. You will be able to attend to and balance out other areas of your life if you engage in activities such as spending quality time with those who matter, engaging in self-care, growing spiritually, dealing with any traumatic or heartbreaking experiences you may have endured in the past, and maintaining a balanced mindset. Because we live in a community comprised of other people, all these aspects of our lives are significant. This implies that we are all susceptible to encountering circumstances and making decisions that will leave us unbalanced in certain aspects of our lives.

Therefore, when you are able to make time for your career and the things that matter, you will experience a sudden surge of fulfillment and joy. This is due to the fact that you will be striving toward wholeness and not just wealth.

Utilize Time Profitably

Using time wisely includes committing to opportunities and events that will flow into you. You must develop the habit of being able to account for every second of your existence in order to see how your time is being spent.

When you prioritize quality over quantity, you will become acutely aware of where you are spending your time. Consequently, if you are scheduled to work 8 hours per day and your time management habits improve, you will want to spend less time on lunch breaks and unnecessary office conversation. Similarly, if you've made it a priority to have family time on the weekends, as your time management skills improve, you'll spend more time interacting with your family instead of believing that it's healthy to be physically present while scrolling through your phone.

Every time you leave an experience, you should feel as though your time was well invested. And each second you account for should contribute to your fulfillment, satisfaction, and happiness. If your commitments cannot deliver this, then you are squandering your time and must begin practicing change in this area.

Conclusion

Time management is life management and an essential entrepreneurial talent. This is an essential resource. Time management is the process of finding methods to work smarter, not harder, in order to complete tasks in less time. Time management can be acquired and must be regularly practiced like any other skill. By learning how to manage your time, you grant yourself the ability to be successful and live a life of your choosing. Due to the number of actions required to develop the skills and the time required to conquer them, it can be difficult to gain control of your time. You will be able to accomplish everything you set out to do with less effort and in less time if you use the techniques and strategies outlined in this book to gain control of your time.

If you can exercise fundamental time management techniques for an extended period of time, your productivity will increase dramatically. Previously unattainable objectives will become more attainable. Previously intimidating duties will no longer appear daunting. Things you never imagined possible will begin to occur if you simply show up and put in the effort.

Time is the next best form of currency, so it is crucial that you utilize it wisely. Learn how to effectively manage your time and you will begin to spend more time doing the activities you enjoy.

After long days of schoolwork, chores, and extracurricular activities, many students are tempted to remain up late because they finally have time to themselves. High school pupils need an average of 8 to 10 hours of sleep per night, according to research conducted by the American Academy of Sleep Medicine. To ensure that your children get adequate slumber, ensure that they:

Incorporate 8 to 10 hours of sleep into their agendas.

Avoid drinking caffeinated beverages before rest.

Stop using electronic devices approximately 30 minutes before the lights are turned out.

Prioritize Important Tasks: When students detest a task, they tend to put it off until the end. Instruct them to begin with the assignment they anticipate to be the most challenging. They will be able to concentrate on their favorite subjects once they have completed the challenging assignments. Have them establish priority by:

Creating to-do lists in a planner and crossing off completed tasks as they are completed.

Estimating a time allotment in advance.

Taking breaks after completing a subject as a reward.

Take Brain Breaks: It may seem counterintuitive, but working continuously is a poor time management habit; students are more productive when they are able to concentrate after sufficient rest. Ensure that they take pauses and have access to nutritious snacks. If you observe a student doing assignments as soon as he or she arrives home, you may want to discuss the student's workload with their instructors. A student who works until late at night and then goes to bed may require tutoring or less assignments.

These are some break-time strategies:

Recharge through brief breaks.

Have a favored snack as a quick reward.

Set a break timer.

Don't Be Afraid to Request Assistance:

Most high school time management skills are designed to foster students' independence, but they also require your assistance to be successful. Sometimes, students hesitate to ask inquiries because they feel like a burden when they need assistance. Inform them that you are available to assist them in completing an assignment or solving a problem.

While assisting them, encourage them to find their own solutions rather than demonstrating how to solve each problem. Permit them to take the lead in homework-related discussions, and encourage them to have confidence in their abilities as you offer suggestions. This way, you're giving them the assistance they require while also teaching them, so they won't have to inquire again in the future.

Some students may feel like they have failed if they deviate from the improvements they had intended to make to their daily routines. For instance, a pupil may take a significantly longer break than what is indicated in their planner. Perceived failures demoralize them, causing them to revert to undesirable behaviors. Ask them to make small, manageable adjustments to their regimen so that they can deviate from it without feeling guilty.

The same concept applies to subpar performance on assignments. Students who receive a lower grade than usual frequently interpret this as evidence that they lack intelligence. Remind them of their past accomplishments, such as winning an award for a research paper they wrote or finishing first in their math class last year. Everyone experiences ups and downs, and a failing grade can be a valuable learning experience if viewed in the proper light.

Chapter 7: Postpone

What are the most common causes for entrepreneurs to return home? Why postpone making a decision, beginning a new project, launching a new business, or concluding a large project that affects multiple businesses?

Here are some justifications.

Walk

• Network contractors have substandard work practices

Typically, handymen with mediocre work ethics are sluggish at everything. They are chronic procrastinators who take an extremely long time to complete a task or endeavor.What may result from this type of net trading?

The loss of commerce and revenue. Deadlines missed and poor communication with buyers and consumers can be detrimental to your business and reputation.

This is not beneficial for the developing Internet and its web entrepreneur.

They constantly attempt to "catch up" with everything else in their lives, including the personal sphere. This results in increased tension and decreased productivity.

Entrepreneurs with subpar work ethics discover that they perform better under pressure. Not truthful.

They believe they produce their finest work when forced to work faster and their creativity is refreshed, but this is not true. All of this delays their work and heightens their tension.

- A constant sense of being overburdened exists.

Web entrepreneurs who struggle with effective time management frequently feel as if they are accomplishing nothing. Frequently unresponsive to working actively or completing duties.

Additionally, overwhelming emotions can cause anxiety and a propensity to make costly errors at work. I'm here. Obviously, this makes the sensation of being overwhelmed and overwhelmed even stronger.

Additionally, there is a feeling of emptiness in business initiatives involving hesitant entrepreneurs. They believe that the size of their business may make doing nothing simpler. Again, this is cyclical and can spiral your business downward. Failure to complete one task can result in the failure of another, with the process continuing and causing additional issues.

• You have the sense that you must be "perfect."

This is likely one of the most prevalent yet most detrimental personality traits among work-at-home entrepreneurs. Worse yet, they must be flawless, avoid errors at all costs, do things correctly the first time, and be able to purposefully meet every desire and requirement of their customers. Not only is this belief unrealistic, but it is also detrimental and unfair for entrepreneurs to hold themselves to this standard. Perfectionism is a delusion for a web entrepreneur. They place undue pressure on themselves to be perfect, despite the fact that it is impossible for them to be so.

They desire to complete assignments, meet deadlines and objectives, and accomplish everything in record time! However, movement is frequently the only thing holding them back.

They may view their business tasks as tedious and avoid them as unimportant. This frequently makes me feel better because it gives me confidence that if I'm not essential, the customer or buyer may not care. Typically, entrepreneurs postpone project completion until maturity standards are met.

Customers typically do not recognize these standards, which are valued only by entrepreneurs. Obviously, this demonstrates that it was a waste of time and unjustly pointed to an unnecessary conclusion.

• Entrepreneurs are Brass Bless? Are DIY enthusiasts truly uninterested? Indeed they do! But this is not the conventional definition of tedium.

They become negligent and their work lacks creativity and innovation. They may enjoy their work, but they find doing the same thing every day tedious and unchallenging. Consequently, you become bored and lose interest in the assignment you are working on.

In many instances, individuals who work from home merely desire to engage in activities other than work. Does this imply they are slothful? Not probable! Frequently, they have no idea where to begin, how to manage a business endeavor, or how to start a business to pursue their own interests.

You can search for alternative, non-business-related techniques such as: B. Instead of doing actual labor, participate in social websites and community discussion forums. Routine duties such as paperwork and Internet work may take precedence over real work.

Entrepreneurs procrastinate with the expectation that the delay will be magically reduced or eliminated. Knowing that this effort is not required increases their level of tension, making tasks more difficult to complete and goals more difficult to attain.

What consequences do these obstacles have? Do you practice effective time management?

Chapter 8: Reduce the use of instantaneous responses

If you have difficulty saying "no," one of the best ways to regain control of your schedule is to stop answering calls immediately. Consider: when asked, we incline to quickly respond with "yes." Then we will be bound into an agreement from which we cannot withdraw. Take a break from the email or politely inform the sender that you need time to consider their question before responding.

Do not make an immediate one-month commitment. Instead, be selective in your commitments and ensure that they align with your values and goals. Be assured in politely declining a request that conflicts with your values and goals. At the conclusion of each month, evaluate your time savings. Your sense of accomplishment and pride may have increased.

BE RESPECTFUL OF YOURSELF

What is the point of attempting to manage your time if you are unwilling to take responsibility for it? Nothing. Suppose you desire to invest more time in your relationship with your significant other and determine to devote one hour per day to providing them with the care and attention they require. Nevertheless, as you wait, your phone begins to vibrate. Therefore, what do you do?

Focus on the person you love and work to develop a stronger, more intense connection with them instead of looking at your phone. By focusing on the ultimate objective and delaying the phone conversation for at least an hour, you can achieve the outcome that best reflects your inner values and will provide you with greater gratification than checking your phone ever could.

Accept accountability for your time management methods.

UTILIZE THE 20-MINUTE RULE, NUMBER NINE

Do you ever feel like you're just...in the zone? You are unstoppable. Imagine being able to enter optimum performance mode at any time. The 20-minute increment block is one of the most effective methods of time management because it enables you to do just that.

Prepare your mind; inform yourself that you are about to pay close attention to something crucial. Prepare for work and set an alarm for twenty minutes from now. Concentrate solely on it until the alarm sounds, and then proceed to the next task. At the sound of the timer, you have the option of abandoning your work or continuing. Put this task on pause while you recharge. Multiple repetitions are required to complete the task.

If you divide your work into 20-minute segments, you can force yourself into the flow state whenever you need it, rather than relying on serendipity. You will eventually be able to attain this state of mind without a timer.

Chapter 9: Tips For Personal Development

There are numerous methods in which we can improve ourselves. Here are a few good ones to begin with, as they may make it easier to work on other aspects of oneself in the future.

Participate in introspection

Self-reflection is an essential component of mindfulness. Without self-reflection, we may not have a reasonable self-concept; that is, our self-concept may not correspond to how others perceive us (Johnson et al., 2002). By engaging in self-reflection, we are more likely to recognize the aspects of ourselves that need improvement and how to work on them. Here you can learn more about self-reflection.

2. Attempt concern

Care is the act of highlighting experience in every moment. It also involves an attitude of curiosity and acknowledgement (rather than judgment) and considering thoughts and emotions to be transient states (Minister et al., 2004). Care, like self-reflection, may make us more receptive to encounters and prospective outcomes that promote personal development.

3. Develop a development outlook

A development outlook is a mentality in which we recognize that we are capable of growth and improvement (Dweck, 2015). If we have a mindset that can be improved, we are obligated to invest the time and effort required to learn and grow. Therefore, developing a development outlook can assist us in achieving a large number of our goals and enhancing ourselves in the ways we desire.

4. acknowledge feelings of disgrace

Cultural tensions (Sedikides and Hepper, 2009), external assumptions, and even shame about insufficiency in a particular area motivate a significant number of individuals to pursue personal development. Nonetheless, if we strive to develop ourselves solely to please others, we are likely to feel dissatisfied regardless of our success in achieving our personal development objectives. Therefore, it is important to consider your motivations for participating in personal development, acknowledge any shame, and reconsider your personal development objectives to ensure they are in accordance with your core values.

Chapter 10: Your Projects Chart

The majority of a company's work comprises of numerous projects. Your professional success is predominantly dependent on your ability to complete projects. A project is defined as multitasking labor. A project is the result of the sequential completion of numerous smaller duties. A checklist is arguably the most effective instrument for enhancing productivity and substantially boosting levels of accomplishment. A checklist is a written inventory of actions in chronological order that is composed prior to beginning work. Your ability to precisely characterize and choose the steps necessary to get from where you are now to a completed project demonstrates your superior intelligence.

By creating protocols and expediting the work completion process, you will save 10 minutes. Another example of how delayed thinking can significantly increase your productivity, effectiveness, and overall company value.

Create a PERT chart.

To assist you and others in understanding your larger activities and initiatives, provide a visual representation. Start by identifying the goals and objectives you must achieve to achieve the desired results. Consider the conclusion before starting. Invest some time in gaining a thorough understanding of what your objectives would entail if they were successfully attained. Then, proceed backwards from the future to the present. Create a list of the logical steps you must take to get from where you are to where you want to be, in that order.

Using a PERT chart, which stands for Program Evaluation Review Technique, you can visualize all of the necessary stages and when they must be completed in order to achieve your ultimate goal. Globally, the most successful businesses and executives employ this strategy. Using a PERT chart, you can see several methods for completing the activity more effectively.

Online, you have access to numerous forms and designs. Figure 1 depicts one illustration. To create the chart, draw a line from the required date of completion for each of your objectives or goals and plot them rearward. Put everything on paper so you can see when you need to complete each assignment stage in order to complete the project on time. When you write down your thoughts and use a PERT chart, you have complete control over the course of events. You are able to run on a track. You may monitor a number of tasks to ensure they are completed on time and up to factory standards. Using a PERT chart will prevent you from becoming overburdened by deadlines. You remain on top of your work and major initiatives.

If you need something completed by the end of the month, you can set your deadline for the fifteenth of the month with plenty of wiggle room or the twentieth of the month, just in case there are unanticipated delays or problems. Murphy's Law states that whatever could go wrong, will go wrong. The dominant executive anticipates problems, obstacles, unanticipated delays, and failures to complete the task by the deadline. These occurrences are prevalent and unavoidable in the business world. It is your responsibility to continuously monitor the project's progress, identify any issues, and then eliminate the inevitable obstacles. However, once you begin using a PERT chart, you may be pleasantly astonished at how much more you can accomplish and how few hiccups or conflicts will occur between the processes.

Establish Everyone's Objectives

Clear, documented objectives for each significant participant in the project will allow you to accomplish more than great conversations and good intentions ever could. Establish time-bound, quantifiable, unambiguous, and specific objectives. Remember that actions are evaluated. Without a deadline, an objective is nothing more than a wish. It is merely a discussion. Each objective or subgoal associated with the completion of a task or project must be assigned to a designated individual. Who will perform this duty? When and to what standard must the assignment be completed?

Always consider these questions. Never assume that others understand your needs until you've made them abundantly obvious.

After enduring massive losses and filing for bankruptcy in 2009, General Motors generated a $4,9 billion profit in 2012. Mr. Dan Akerson, According to the President of GM, the most crucial aspect of the company's recovery was the formulation of specific objectives for each key individual and at every level of the business. Before assuming the position, he discovered that the organization's goals were typically vague, unclear, unenforced, and infrequently achieved. After establishing clearly defined goals, all employees were aware of what was required of them to advance their careers and retain their jobs.

Remember that your capacity for thought, especially your capacity for anticipatory thought, is your most remarkable ability. The more time you devote to deliberation and the creation of a written plan, the better and more quickly you will achieve your goals.

1.2 The Value of Time Administration

Time management is essential because it allows you to plan your day in order to expand your business while maintaining a healthy work-life balance. The advantages of effective time management are as follows:

You will have a better understanding of what you must do and how long each task should take if you learn to schedule time during the week for many of your essential responsibilities. When you adhere to a schedule, you will likely spend less time deciding what to focus on or delaying tasks and more time getting things done. Time management allows you to focus on the most important duties while avoiding time-consuming distractions.

If you were not constantly rushing to achieve a deadline, you could concentrate more on your work. Multitasking allows you to prioritize your assignments and ensure you have sufficient time to complete each one. The quality of work improves, but only if there is sufficient time to meet deadlines.

If you want to effectively manage your time, give each item on your agenda its own time slot. Numerous individuals make efficient use of their time by allowing themselves many days to complete a task or by beginning it earlier than required to account for unforeseen obstacles. If you accurately estimate the time required to complete a task, you will always achieve your objectives.

If you are able to effectively manage company time and meet deadlines, you will feel fulfilled and confident in your abilities. Regularly removing items from your daily to-do list is a powerful motivator that may encourage individuals to improve their time management and seek out new employment opportunities. When objectives are accomplished, a sense of satisfaction may ensue. For instance, they may resolve to complete a task by Friday in order to spend the weekend catching up with coworkers.

By effectively managing their time, students can complete their assignments on time, remain engaged in their studies, and have more time for activities that are essential to them, such as sports, youth group, and spending time with friends and family.

Students can enhance their time management with the help of a variety of strategies.

Plan Your Launch

Develop a production schedule to set aside time for studies or project work. Determine the duration of each procedure to determine how much time to allot daily or weekly. Make an effort to study every workday, even if only for a brief period. The timeline can be made easier to comprehend by color-coding particular topics.

Prepare initiatives.

When studying or duties appear challenging, procrastination is common. Your child's research proposal or assignment should be divided into smaller, more manageable portions. You could provide a deadline to encourage each component to reach its small objectives.

Given all of these benefits, it seems reasonable to conclude that planning has been one of the keys to improved work outcomes, professional advancement, and a happier, more fulfilled life. Understanding how time managers function and using them effectively requires effort, but this method makes it easier to deal with the turmoil of modern life. But the long-term value of time management outweighs the dangers and difficulties of learning.

What function does it serve in our lives?

Time management benefits include enhanced habits and increased productivity. Effective time management improves your disposition, concentration, and schedule. Small business owners, artisans, and entrepreneurs can reap the benefits of effective time management. Time management skills enhance job satisfaction and work-life balance. In addition to reducing tension, effective time management facilitates the accomplishment of one's objectives. Time management is essential in numerous facets of your existence. It is necessary for increased productivity and improved prioritization. Additionally, meeting deadlines motivates you to organize your time more carefully. Time management enables you to work wiser, not harder, complete more in less time, and seize more opportunities.

The advantages of time management are evident. Time management skills enable you to accomplish more in less time through greater time flexibility, enhanced concentration, increased creativity, reduced tension, and more time spent with loved ones who are more important to you. When you effectively manage your time, greater outcomes and more consequential decisions are inevitable. In addition to increased productivity and efficiency, time management also reduces tension. Workplace time management that is effective involves working less and accomplishing more.

These strategies enhance your performance and focus. Additionally, they reduce interruptions and complacency. You will be more productive if you manage your time through effective project planning. Additionally, it allows you to complete more essential tasks.

Reduce stress

Time management and meeting deadlines are two examples of effective scheduling. Controlling your schedule will prevent you from experiencing chronic tension and fatigue. If you effectively manage your time, you may be even more productive. You are able to manage your workload and prioritize the most essential tasks due to your increased productivity. You feel more assured and less anxious about how to spend your time. Manage the pressures that hinder your time management skills. Determine the causes of your tension and the effects its elimination would have.

More personal leisure

One of the greatest benefits of time management is having more time flexibility. When you have sufficient leisure, you can set and achieve your most important objectives. You've had significantly more time to investigate new interests and hone existing ones. Greater temporal adaptability allows you to accomplish your ultimate objective. Consider the potential changes that may occur to the three most essential items. Create a detailed action plan to put these changes into effect.

A Greater Degree of Concentration

Effective time management boosts your memory and concentration. By giving things more consideration, you may be able to seize more opportunities. Additionally, it allows you to focus more on the initiatives, objectives, and people that are most important to you. When you manage your time, you can better organize your day and improve your performance. Having a daily plan increases efficiency. Time management necessitates planning your activities.

Chapter 11: If You Cannot Consume It All, Do Not Consume It.

Occasionally, we take on more than we can handle. I have committed this offense far too frequently to enumerate. We want to do everything, and we want to do it immediately, genuinely believing that we can accomplish everything if we just plan our time efficiently.

Unfortunately, however, this is not always the case. Life is unpredictable and can derail us utterly. Our painting day must be postponed because our great-uncle is in town and wants to have lunch. Everything we do seems to take twice as long as anticipated because we awake congested as heck and seemingly moving in slow motion. Or, we must miss a day of work because our roof was damaged by a tempest and requires repair; it could be anything.

Due to our relative lack of ESP, we cannot precisely predict these events, but we can prevent them from being too catastrophic when they do occur.

The best method to accomplish this, and to eliminate a great deal of stress, is to avoid attempting to do too much in too little time. Do not schedule your day to the minute. Instead, you should ensure that you have a small buffer of time.

Since we can write 1,000 words per hour, we might believe that writing 7,000 words per day is perfectly feasible, correct? Well, if you get sidetracked or spend more time researching a topic than anticipated, you could wind up writing approximately 4,000 words in one day. Since you've set a daily goal of 7,000 words, you'll have to write 10,000 words tomorrow, which is highly improbable. You'll be continually playing catch-up, and, spoiler alert, you'll never catch up, at least not on time.

Be realistic in your goal-setting. Even if it's possible to write 7,000 words per day, and even if you've done it before, you must realize that if you continue to press yourself and hold yourself to these unreasonable standards every single day, you'll burn out. Not only will it be detrimental to you and your health, but it will also have a negative impact on the work you've been pressing yourself so hard for.

Consider the repercussions of not taking action. Consider what would occur if a task is either not completed in full or not completed on time. Who will be impacted? Will the residence continue to be slightly unclean for another week? Or is it something like your coworkers being unable to progress forward until you've completed your tasks? As an enjoyable psychological bonus, the fear of disappointing others is a powerful motivator. Not optimal, but functional.

This does kind of fall under the umbrella of determining the importance of your tasks when organizing them, but I wanted to add it here because if you are overwhelmed by certain tasks — or too many tasks — then weighing the consequences of not doing them can help you determine whether you can drop a particular task entirely or simply postpone it temporarily.

When you need support, do not be afraid to ask for it. Many people find it extremely difficult to seek for assistance because it feels like a sign of failure. However, as I mentioned previously, pushing yourself too hard will only result in burnout, and your work and life will suffer as a result.

Asking for assistance could involve asking someone to assist you with a task, but it could also involve requesting a deadline extension or ordering takeout instead of cooking to save time. A small amount of assistance from another person or a small amount of extra time can be extremely beneficial and prevent us from pulling out our hair.

Be courteous to yourself. You are your greatest asset, so establish objectives that you can achieve without exhausting yourself in the process.

Chapter 12: Record The Tasks That Must Be Completed Today

There is nothing more demotivating than having an excessively long list of tasks. Instead of listing multiple projects on a single, massive to-do list, create separate lists for each project and assign time limits to each task.

To accomplish today's tasks efficiently and effectively, you should first write them down. Once you've completed that list (or if it's a larger endeavor or objective), write down tomorrow's tasks. Then, proceed to the following week or month. This will help you focus on your daily objectives so you don't burn out soon, and it will also provide direction for future objectives and tasks.

Remember that any task that can be completed in less than 5 minutes should not be listed. These items readily fit into your immediate to-do list Now Record Tomorrow's Assignments: The initial step toward achieving your objectives is to break them down into actionable actions. To move things forward, schedule time throughout the day to work on these steps, even if they are minor. Before going to bed at the conclusion of every single day, write down the tasks that must be completed the following day.

By putting yourself in future mode the night before you go to sleep, you will already know where to focus your energy for maximal productivity throughout the day when you open your journal the next morning. So far, we have discussed daily task management and planning for tomorrow. What about long-term planning, though? How do I plan for the future? Personal and professional long-term planning entails establishing quarterly, yearly, and lifetime objectives, and then working backwards to determine the actions you must take right now to reach those objectives. While some people prefer to use Excel or Google Sheets for long-term planning, others prefer pen and paper because it is simpler to modify as circumstances change.

When planning your long-term objectives, keep in mind that it is essential to consider big while remaining practical. It's easy to feel overwhelmed by big ideas, but if you break them down into smaller pieces, you'll feel more motivated and inspired as you move forward. Your Greatest Objectives Should Motivate You: When considering your major life objectives, ask yourself the following two questions:

1) Why am I performing this action?

2) How will my existence be enhanced?

once I achieve my objective? Let's say that one of your greatest career aspirations is to be promoted within six months. Consider why you want the promotion and how it would affect your life if you received it. Perhaps you desire a promotion because earning more money would enable you to purchase your own home.

Perhaps you desire a promotion because it would result in more vacation days, allowing you to travel abroad. Perhaps you desire a promotion because it would boost your confidence and enable you to pursue other objectives. Whatever your reasons are for desiring that promotion, they will serve as your inspiration and motivation. In fact, if that promotion does not stimulate or inspire you in some way, it may not even be worth pursuing.

When defining your long-term objectives, you should always consider the why and the impact that attaining the objective will have on your life.

Chapter 13: Before You Begin

At the outset of my journey, I did not comprehend this region, which limited my ability to become genuinely useful. Consequently, I cannot accept your assessment of this region on the same basis. In order to rectify my oversight, I've compiled a list of the prerequisite knowledge you must have before beginning.

First, I want you to know that I recognize you as a self-motivated individual.

I believe you will achieve prosperity.

I understand that you are doing this because you have a goal to achieve. I accept, above all, that you obtain what is significant in your existence.

I am referring to a fundamental understanding of the primary role you perform in the area where you hope to be useful.

This is the fundamental building block to becoming more useful in ordinary life. You MUST recognize the actions that produce the most significant outcomes. Whether you are an employee or an entrepreneur, you must recognize the most valuable aspects of your employment. This is such an important point that I should write an entire volume about it.

This is your area of influence.

Your area of influence (AOI) is your primary influence at work. By devoting more time and effort to this, you will produce more results and get closer to your goals more quickly than if you did anything else.

I struggled with this aspect of my existence for quite a while. I would work for prolonged periods under the impression that I was achieving a great deal, but in general I am wasting my resources. This is a small window of opportunity during the day, and your objective is to maximize results with the time available. Only after some time had passed did I realize that by focusing on my area of influence, I could considerably increase my results in the same amount of time.

One query is sufficient to reveal your AOI, regardless of what you do. The question is, "What do I do that has the greatest impact on?" If you are a representative, you should ask your superior, "What do I do in my position that significantly impacts the company?"

Additional questions may include: Which responsibilities are most crucial to your job? What are the most important indicators of whether you are dominant in your position?

The responses may surprise you.

If you are self-employed, ask yourself the same questions, but in the context of your business.

An additional line addressing the right: What metrics indicate the business is expanding? What duties contribute to this growth? What roles do you perform in these activities?

When I first conceived of the concept of AOI, I believed that each individual had a unique AOI. In addition to having an AOI for your career, you also have an AOI for every significant aspect of your existence. This encompasses relationships, family, otherworldliness, happiness, and general life satisfaction. There is something you do in each of these areas that produces the majority of your results.

For the benefit of your relationship, it may be necessary to invest quality time with your significant other.

Quite possibly, Sunday dinner is a weekly tradition for your family. Depending on your otherworldliness, you may require 20 minutes per day to reconnect.

It may very well be submitting random acts of thoughtfulness each day for your pleasure.

Your desired week may be one step closer, much to your satisfaction. You should be able to see where I'm going with this. Everyone has a unique AOI, and only you will know what yours is. It is not enigmatic. Collectively, we have a good understanding of what has the greatest impact on our existence. All that is required is a little self-reflection and a guarantee to zero in on it.

This is the essential key to becoming more effective, as 80% of this book is derived from it. Towards the end of the book, we will discuss additional techniques for the most effective execution of your AOI, but until then, you need to have a clever idea.

Chapter 14: Concentrating On Mental Health Through Meditation

The most well-known and well-documented benefit of meditation is an increase in tranquility. This increased tranquility can help you experience a variety of health benefits and enhance your stress-management skills. When you are able to manage tension more effectively, you can reduce your heart rate, blood pressure, and cortisol levels. Meditation practice in the morning can help you focus your mind and body and unwind before you begin your daily routine. If you are stressed about projects, clients, deadlines, or other aspects of your business, meditating can help you forget about these issues before you begin your day.

Meditation can also help you achieve a healthier life balance and avoid exhaustion. Many people, including entrepreneurs, believe that you must labor sixteen hours per day to launch and maintain a successful business. Long-term success necessitates balancing your work with other aspects of your life, despite the fact that building a successful business requires hard labor and commitment.

It is more probable that burnout will contribute to failure. However, maintaining a balance in your life can contribute to your success, not only in your career but in other areas as well. The greater your time management skills, the more time you will have to take care of yourself mentally and physically, thereby preventing exhaustion.

2. MAINTAIN TO-DO-LIST

Do you frequently feel overwhelmed by the amount of work you must complete, or do you frequently miss deadlines? Or do you sometimes forget to do something important, prompting your supervisor to remind you to complete your tasks?

All of these are consequences of not maintaining an adequate "To-Do List." These are prioritized lists of all the tasks you must complete. Theu list everything that you have to do, with the most important tasks listed first and the least important tasks listed last.

By keeping a journal, you ensure that your assignments are written down in a single location so you don't forget anything important. Also, by prioritizing tasks, you plan the order in which you'll complete them, allowing you to determine which tasks require immediate attention and which can wait.

To-Do Lists are essential if you want to avoid work overload. You will appear unfocused and unreliable to the people around you if you fail to utilize them effectively.

When you utilize them efficiently, you will be much more organized and reliable. You will experience less stress knowing that you have not forgotten anything crucial. In addition, if you prioritize intelligently, you will focus your time and energy on high-value activities, which will make you more useful and valuable to your team.

Keeping an appropriately trustured and well-considered list sounds mrle. However, it is shocking how many individuals fail to use them at all, let alone effectively.

In fast, it is frequently when individuals begin to use them efficiently and effectively that they achieve their first professional breakthrough and begin to achieve success in their careers. This video explains how to begin using To-Do List more efficiently.

Step 1: Write down all of the tasks you must complete. Assuming they are substantial endeavors, separate the first assignment from the larger project. (Ideally, duties or ascension steps should not take more than one to two hours to complete.)

You may find it simpler to organize multiple lt (encompassing personal, academic, and professional topics). Truly unique arrroashe and use the best for your situation.

Step 2 : Run through these tasks in order of importance or urgency, beginning with the most important or urgent and ending with the least important or least urgent.

If a large number of tak have a high rrortu, re-examine the list and demote the less significant ones. After completing this, revise the list's rrortu order.

Deal with the A rrortu tak first, followed by the Bs, the Cs, and so on, in order to utilize your list. As you complete errands, check them off or complete them.

What you write on your list and how you use it depends on your situation. For example, if you are in a leadership role, one way to motivate yourself is to keep your to-do list short and aim to complete it each day.

But if you're in a managerial position, or if your responsibilities involve a large number of people, it may be preferable to fosu on a longer-term list and "shr awau" at it.

Many roles find it beneficial to spend 10 minutes at the end of the day organizing their tasks for the following day.

Chapter 15: Utilizing Time Management

Improve Study Skills

The majority of students begin each new semester with high expectations. They believe they will be successful in their studies and schoolwork, but they fail to create a realistic plan or establish a regimen that will allow them to achieve academic success. There are a limited number of hours per day, days per week, and weeks per term. And if you're not careful, the conclusion of the semester will sneak up on you, catching you by surprise. To attain academic success, you must manage your daily, weekly, and semester study time with precision. The following is a time management strategy for achieving this specific objective.

Step 1. Prepare a Term Calendar

At the beginning of each new term, before you become heavily engaged in your studies or other activities, create an all-term calendar. Your term calendar may resemble a standard monthly calendar or have a distinctive layout. Regardless of the format chosen, your term calendar should include the following:

responsibilities with due deadlines

Tests with their respective periods

All academic pursuits

All extracurricular and extramural activities

Step 2: Create a weekly calendar

In contrast to your term calendar, which is plotted out in full at the beginning of each term, your weekly schedule is created at the start of each week. every Sunday Prepare a weekly schedule by settling down. Although you will prepare your weekly schedule every Sunday, you should update it as new items arise throughout the week. To prepare your weekly schedule, follow the steps below:

Record each class you have each day of the week on your calendar.

Take a look at your term calendar and jot down on your weekly calendar items that need to be completed or are occurring that week (i.e., assignments, tests, events, etc.).

Review your class notes and last week's schedule to determine if there is anything you need to add to this week's schedule.

Include in your weekly schedule any extracurricular and non-school activities that you will be participating in during the forthcoming week.

Notate the date and time of each assignment, study session, work group, and project that you will complete during the week. These could take place in the evening, after school, or during the school day.

Step 3: Plan your daily activities

You may believe that a term calendar and weekly schedule are sufficient for time management, but they are not. Additionally, you must create a daily schedule. Prepare a daily schedule for the next school day each night. Place a checkmark next to each completed task as it is accomplished. To create your daily timetable, complete the steps below:

Write down everything from your weekly timetable that must be completed tomorrow.

Notate the unfinished tasks from the previous day's agenda that must be completed the following day.

Check your daily timetable for the current day to see if you need to add any additional school activities for the following day.

Include any additional activities from your weekly timetable that need to be incorporated into tomorrow's agenda.

One of the keys to effectively managing your study time is to start with the broad picture and work your way down to the specifics. Your term calendar provides instruction and direction for achieving the overall objective. Your daily and weekly schedules provide the necessary detail to execute everything on your term calendar, allowing you to achieve your term objectives one day and one week at a time.

Chapter 16: Ensure You Complete Your Assignments

Some individuals accept more work than they are capable of completing, while others accept assignments without the intention of completing them. Both scenarios are unsatisfactory and extremely detrimental, and neither is a desirable behavior.

Finished Tasks

The initial step in addressing this issue is determining one's competence and suitability for the task at hand. When evaluating a task and deciding to undertake it, the initial attitude must be both positive and open.

With the correct mentality at the outset of a task, the initial obstacle is successfully surmounted. Attitude plays a significant role in determining whether the task will be completed and whether the results will be satisfactory.

It is also advisable to provide a timeline for the completion of a mission. This timeline should ideally be realistic and realizable. When this truth about the schedule is explicitly and firmly enshrined in the task framework, everyone can focus on completing the assignment.

Developing the mindset and discipline of completing one task before moving on to the next is crucial. Every undertaking should have a system of checks and balances to ensure that it runs smoothly. It also contributes to a feeling of accomplishment when each task is accomplished successfully. Both the task supervisor and the participant's confidence will increase, resulting in the establishment of a positive reputation. The efficiency with which a person completes a mission demonstrates that he or she is reliable and trustworthy. Once these firm work ethics have been established, it is possible to assign additional tasks with confidence.

Chapter 17: Utilize Self-Affirmations To Conquer Procrastination

Although there are numerous instruments available to help people motivate themselves, there is no substitute for intrinsic motivation.

Listening to numerous motivational speeches, reading motivational literature, acquiring motivational skills, or even being surrounded by highly motivated individuals may not always be sufficient to inspire someone to go the extra mile. This is something the individual must accomplish independently. Individually and with conviction, a positive decision must be made.

Several Recommendations

Numerous individuals have attested that self-motivation is effective when applied accurately and consistently. The effectiveness of overcoming procrastination is enhanced by a constant barrage of positive self-talk or inspiration.

When no one else is available to encourage you, self-talk is the next best thing. Repeating a few straightforward optimistic concepts and captions over and over again can "trick" the mind into accepting them as true, thereby making it easy to overcome procrastination.

When this "truth" is thoroughly embraced and incorporated into an individual's thinking, the war against procrastination is nearly won. The train and the incline is the most popular, and some might even say ridiculous, but effective line that many people use. It goes I believe in myself, I believe in myself. Here are some additional self-talk phrases recommended for overcoming procrastination:

• I can do it; I'll do it; I'm doing it; I want to do it; I'm a success; I'm a capable individual; I'll succeed.

Chapter 18: Effective Objective Setting

Setting objectives is essential for operating a successful business, whether it's an online e-commerce store or a brick-and-mortar store. Everyone will interpret goal-setting differently. But what is goal setting exactly, and are you doing it correctly?

Simply put, goal setting is the process of developing an action plan to help you achieve the objective you've set. It begins with identifying your objectives, followed by a description of the actions you will take to achieve them. Let's examine the fundamentals of goal setting and offer guidance on how to use this effective performance strategy to boost employee commitment, motivation, and overall productivity.

Multiple studies have demonstrated that setting objectives increases productivity and quality. Psychiatrists Gary Latham and Edwin

Locke assert that establishing goals can increase productivity by 11 to 25 percent. In today's global workplace, productivity is more important than ever.

Many individuals are either completely goalless or extremely goal-oriented. People without objectives tend to drift through life, oblivious to why they aren't completely satisfied. Although they may (or may not) attain monetary success, goal-oriented people are rarely content, as they are constantly under duress. Finding a comfortable medium in terms of goal-setting is essential for achieving life satisfaction and harmony.

Some individuals are satisfied with merely having a sense of "direction" in their lives, but this can lead to impulsive and reactive behavior in the (often futile) pursuit of a greater sense of fulfillment. However, these individuals frequently realize late in life that they have missed out on all of life's pleasures.

Alternatively, if you only focus on your goals, you may discover that you are the type of person who is always searching for a new goal to motivate you, but without a goal, you will feel restless and aimless. No matter how many goals you accomplish, you will never be content because "the grass is always greener." You must proceed to the next destination because you believe it will increase your happiness. Nevertheless, you must question yourself, "When will I be HAPPY?" If you identify with this, you are likely someone who never appreciates the journey or even relishes a victory by focusing on the present. They are already considering their next objective activity, and they never appear to appreciate the journey or the outcome. This is the experience of goal-oriented individuals.

4.1 Why is Goal Setting So Important?

We are aware of the importance of having goals, but we frequently overlook their significance throughout our lives. Setting goals can assist you in forming new habits, focusing your attention, and maintaining your forward momentum.

Goals can also help you concentrate and feel more in charge. You cannot manage what you do not evaluate, and you cannot expand what you do not effectively control. Setting goals can help you accomplish all of these duties and more. Additionally, we will examine how setting objectives can help you achieve better results. Setting goals can improve our mental health as well as our professional and personal achievements. On our paths to success, it is impossible to overstate the importance of goal-setting. This is why there is so much information available on SMART objectives and why institutions teach this skill to some extent.

Learning the value of wise goals and the benefits of adhering to them will determine whether we value goal setting or not. If we adopt this strategy, we have a much greater chance of achieving our personal and professional objectives.

Our Objectives Guide Our Focus.

If you don't know what you want to accomplish in life, it will be difficult to get there. Some individuals appear to believe that ignoring goals will result in a happier existence. How often have you heard the expression, "I can't be dissatisfied if I have no goals"?

However, is this the conclusion of our story, or can you make some adjustments? Do you wish to exist in order to avoid disappointment?

Without objectives, we lack direction and clarity. Managing expectations is possible, but it does not guarantee pleasure. If we do not have objectives, we will waste time, effort, and energy. Every expert in their field will tell you the same thing: "Yes, talent matters, but what you do with it matters even more."

And your focus determines how you utilize your talent.

Your goals serve as a compass. Your objectives provide you with a destination to strive for. This mental guidance and target will prevent you from straying from your most important life objectives. These objectives will help you align your activities and behaviors as you progress.

What is the significance of establishing goals? It provides you with significance, purpose, and consistency! Many of us have elevated objectives and aspirations. It is among the fascinating facets of our existence!

However, many of us rarely contemplate how to efficiently travel from A to B. Consequently, we rarely achieve these objectives completely. We gaze at our objectives and realize that only a small percentage of people achieve them, so we conclude that we are unqualified for that level of success. Observing the completed product of a goal can be terrifying and deter us from attaining it.

Fortunately, goal setting allows us to break down enormous, terrifying tasks into more manageable ones. These small steps and attainable objectives will help us obtain momentum and encourage us to continue working toward the next phase of our objective.

Regardless of our aspirations, they establish the groundwork for us to begin creating the life we want for ourselves, our families, and even our nations!